HOLLY CEFREY

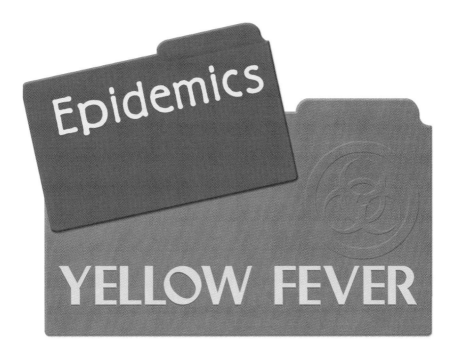

Epidemics

YELLOW FEVER

The Rosen Publishing Group, Inc.
New York

Published in 2002 by The Rosen Publishing Group, Inc.
29 East 21st Street, New York, NY 10010

Library of Congress Cataloging-in-Publication Data

Cefrey, Holly.
Yellow fever / by Holly Cefrey.— 1st ed.
p. ; cm. — (Epidemics)
Includes bibliographical references and index.
ISBN 0-8239-3489-6 (library binding)
1. Yellow fever—Juvenile literature. [1. Yellow fever.
2. Epidemics. 3. Mosquitoes as carriers of disease. 4. Diseases.]
[DNLM: 1. Yellow Fever—History—Popular Works. WC 532
C389y 2002]
I. Title. II. Series.
RA644.Y4 C375 2002

2001001865

Cover image: An electron micrograph of yellow fever viruses.

Manufactured in the United States of America

CONTENTS

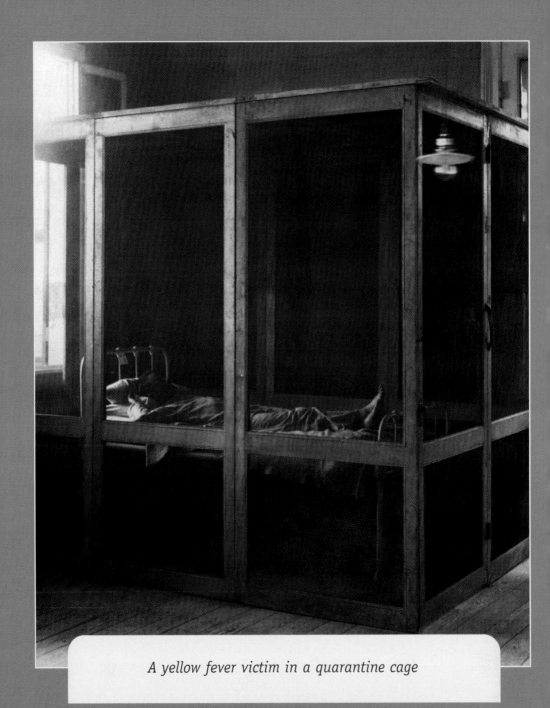

A yellow fever victim in a quarantine cage

INTRODUCTION

The sickness that we feared struck home. My brother Jonathan came down with the fever, and before I knew it, he was barely clinging to life. It all happened very quickly.

The whites of his eyes and his skin turned yellow. We had heard about this yellow sickness but didn't think that we would catch it. So far, only the people who lived in the city were getting sick, and we lived in the country where it was clean and safe. Somehow, it found its way to us.

My brother screamed in agony. With great force, he threw up what looked like black mud. He could not stop vomiting, and it left him weak with exhaustion.

Jonathan looked horrible. His skin became more and more yellow, and his lips cracked and started to ooze blood. He also bled from his nose and mouth. It was as if his insides were changing him into a different being.

Our doctor said that there was nothing he could do for Jonathan . . . that he might get better, or he might not. It was terrible to sit by and watch him in such pain. A few days after the doctor's visit, my brother passed away. For some unknown reason, the rest of my family didn't get sick. We somehow avoided the yellow sickness even though it was in our own home. We live in fear that it may return.

—Fiona, 1811

The disease that took Jonathan's life is called yellow fever. It is a disease that has caused hundreds of epidemics, or outbreaks of disease, in areas all over the world. Outbreaks of yellow fever were common during the seventeenth, eighteenth, and nineteenth centuries. Many large cities, including Boston, New Orleans, and New York were ravaged by the disease on a number of occasions.

People around the world lived in fear of yellow fever. Even worse, the cause of the disease was

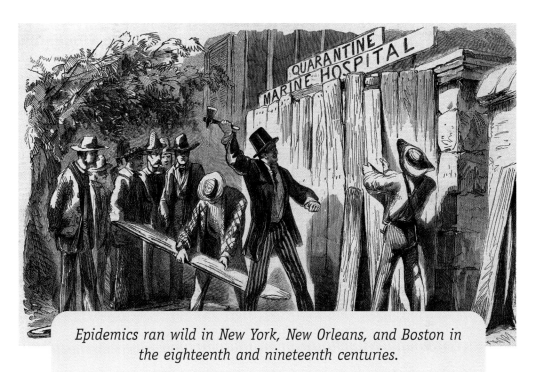
Epidemics ran wild in New York, New Orleans, and Boston in the eighteenth and nineteenth centuries.

unknown. Many doctors believed that the disease was caused by the dirty conditions in large cities. They believed that rotting animal carcasses and human waste, which often littered the streets, were the sources of the disease. It was not until 1900 that doctors discovered the real cause of yellow fever.

Although outbreaks of yellow fever do not make front-page news as they did in the past, the disease still exists in many parts of the world. The World Health Organization (WHO) estimates that 200,000 cases of yellow fever occur each year around the globe. Out of those 200,000 cases, an estimated 30,000 result in death.

1

WHAT IS YELLOW FEVER?

Yellow fever is a disease that is caused by a virus. A virus is a microorganism. A microorganism is a very small, living thing. A microorganism is so small that it cannot be seen without the assistance of a very powerful microscope. Viruses cause sickness and disease, ranging from the common cold to life-threatening illnesses such as AIDS.

The virus that causes yellow fever comes from a family of viruses called flaviviridae. A virus from the flaviviridae family is also called a flavivirus. According to the World Health Organization, there are over seventy different types of flaviviruses in the world.

The World of a Virus

Viruses cannot live on their own. They need to be inside of another organism in order to survive. Humans, animals, plants, and even bacteria are organisms that can become infected with viruses. Organisms that viruses infect are called hosts.

Viruses are very tiny particles that exist all around us. Virus particles in our environment can be found in the air, on the surfaces of objects, and in other living organisms. An individual virus particle is called a virion. A virion can find a host in a number of ways. Two common ways that a virus enters a host are through air passageways, such as the nose and mouth, and through openings in the skin, such as cuts or scrapes.

All virions have something in common: Each must find a cell within a host in order to multiply. A cell is a very small part of a body. A host's body, such as a human's body, is filled with over 200 different types of cells. Each virion looks for a particular kind of cell to become its host cell. A typical flu virion will target the cells of the digestive system (stomach and intestines) or the respiratory system (nasal cavity and lungs). The yellow fever virion targets the cells of the immune system (lymph nodes, spleen, and bone marrow) as well as the cells of the liver, kidneys, and digestive tract.

Once the virion has found a host cell, the virion attaches itself to the cell. The cell becomes the host as new viruses are made within the cell. The new viruses multiply by using the cell's resources. Soon there are so many new virus particles that they burst out of the cell. Once outside, the new viruses start attacking other cells. In this way, the virus spreads throughout the host's body.

Just as viruses look for certain cells, they also look for certain hosts. Hosts are divided into three kingdoms—animal, plant, and bacteria. Many viruses infect the hosts of only one kingdom. The yellow fever virus infects the animal kingdom, which includes humans. The main hosts for the yellow fever virus are humans and primates, which include apes and monkeys.

The Yellow Fever Virus at Work

The yellow fever virus multiplies itself more quickly in areas of the world where the weather is warm. The most agreeable climate for the virus is that of the tropics. The tropics are located near the equator of the earth. In a tropical climate, warm temperatures occur throughout the year. The yellow fever virus

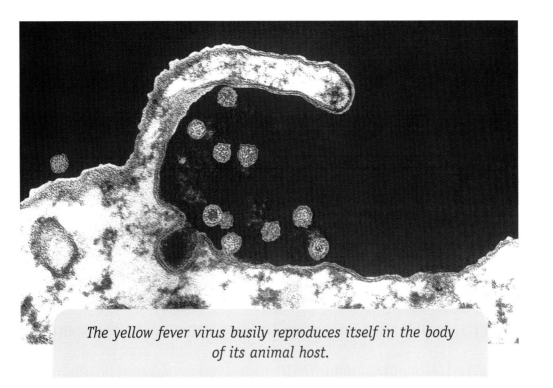

The yellow fever virus busily reproduces itself in the body of its animal host.

thrives in the favorable climates of South and Central America, and Africa.

Yellow fever is transmitted, or spread, to hosts by a vector. A vector is an insect or other organism that is infected with, carries, and spreads a disease. The main vector for yellow fever is the mosquito.

Mosquitoes

Since mosquitoes are most active in warm temperatures, they thrive in the tropics. In areas of the world where parts of the year are cold, mosquitoes cannot survive through the cold season. In the warm winter seasons of the tropics, mosquitoes can hibernate or rest, rather than die. The ability to hibernate increases the life span of mosquitoes.

In addition to being warm, the tropics also have long rainy seasons. Mosquitoes must lay their eggs in pools of water, so the moist climate of the tropics gives mosquitoes many places to breed. The combination of warm weather and moist conditions in the tropics provides an ideal breeding ground for mosquitoes.

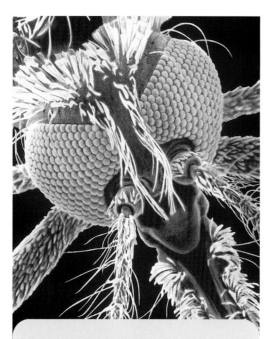

Mosquitoes are the main vector for spreading yellow fever.

Infection in Mosquitoes

Mosquitoes drink the nectar, or juice, of plants as their main source of food. Sometimes, however, female mosquitoes will drink the blood of animals for food. If a blood-drinking mosquito lives in an area where the yellow fever virus has infected animals, the mosquito can spread yellow fever further. The mosquito will bite an infected host. The blood from the infected host, which has the yellow fever virus in it, will be drawn into the mosquito. The mosquito is then infected by the virus and will spread the yellow fever virus to the next host that it bites.

The infected mosquito can pass the yellow fever virus on to animals and people for the rest of its life (as long as eight months). This means that the mosquito is able to infect many hosts over the course of its life. Infected mosquitoes often pass the virus on to their offspring as well. The eggs that the mosquito lays will be infected with the yellow fever virus. When the eggs hatch, the new mosquitoes will be carrying the virus.

The Transmission of Yellow Fever

Transmission of the yellow fever virus happens when the virus is passed from one host to another. There are two main types of transmission: jungle transmission and urban transmission. Jungle transmission occurs in tropical rain forests or jungles. Urban transmission occurs in villages, towns, and cities. A third type of transmission, called intermediate, is a combination of jungle and urban transmission.

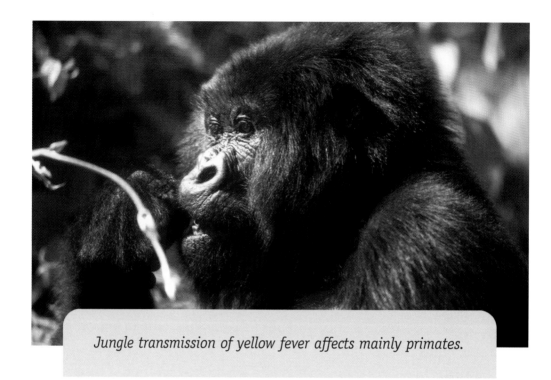

Jungle transmission of yellow fever affects mainly primates.

Jungle Transmission

Jungle transmission affects mainly primates (monkeys and apes). Mosquitoes bite infected primates and then spread the disease by biting other primates. This disease exists as a part of the natural cycle of the rain forest.

When there are no primate hosts present, the yellow fever virus can still exist in the mosquito population. The virus survives in hibernating mosquitoes or in the offspring of infected mosquitoes until hosts are found. Mosquitoes that are hatched with the disease are also responsible for jungle transmission.

Jungle transmission usually involves the spread of the virus from primate to primate. It can, however, spread from primate to human. This happens when humans accidentally become involved in the cycle. Humans who travel to or work in tropical forests can get bitten by infected mosquitoes. Once bitten, the humans become hosts to the virus and suffer its effects.

Urban Transmission

Urban transmission affects mainly humans. The *Aedes aegypti* mosquito, which lives among human populations, is the main vector in urban transmission. Infected mosquitoes spread the disease among human populations.

Urban transmission involves the spread of the virus from human to human. Epidemics can occur when an infected person from one city travels to another city and is bitten by a mosquito. The mosquito can then spread the disease to anyone else that it bites.

Intermediate Transmission

Intermediate transmission affects both primates and humans. Intermediate transmission occurs in areas where urban populations are close to tropical forests. Mosquitoes from both areas can spread the disease from primate to human, or from human to primate.

Yellow fever has been a part of human history for more than three hundred years. During this time, the fever has been known by a few different names.

- *Yellow Jack*—The word "jack" is a nautical, or sailing, term. A jack is a flag that is displayed on a ship's mast, or pole. Ships display flags to be identified by other sea voyagers and by people on shore. Ships that carried people infected with yellow fever were required to hoist a yellow flag as a warning. Ships with yellow flags were quarantined for forty days in port harbors.

- *Vomito Negro*—The Spanish called yellow fever by this name, which means black vomit. A classic symptom of yellow fever is the vomiting of blood that has collected in the stomach and been turned black by stomach acids.

Yellow Fever Infection

The effects of yellow fever can range from mild illness to death. In mild cases, patients may experience fever, chills, headache, backache, and muscle pain. The patient may also experience nausea and vomiting. These signs of infection are called symptoms.

According to the World Health Organization, about 15 percent of patients infected with yellow fever will develop serious infections. In serious infections,

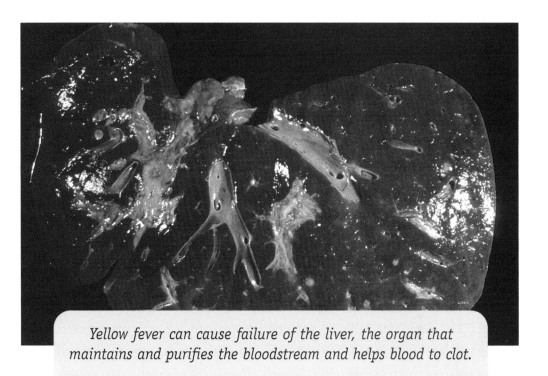

Yellow fever can cause failure of the liver, the organ that maintains and purifies the bloodstream and helps blood to clot.

symptoms progress to jaundice, liver failure, hemor-rhaging, and kidney failure. These symptoms are considered to be the toxic, or poisonous, phase of yellow fever. The World Health Organization estimates that at least half of the patients who reach the toxic phase do not survive.

Yellow fever takes its name from the yellow color that appears on the skin and in the eyes of seriously infected people. This yellowing of the skin is called jaundice, and it is a sign of liver failure. Liver failure takes place when the liver is no longer functioning properly. The proper functioning of the liver is necessary for survival because the liver is responsible for maintaining and purifying the blood.

The liver also plays a key role in helping our blood to clot. Because of this, liver failure often leads to hemorrhaging. Hemorrhaging is the discharging of blood in large amounts. This includes bleeding from the mouth, the nose, the stomach, the rectum, and recent cuts or scrapes. Blood also collects in the stomach. The vomiting of this blood, which is turned black by stomach acids, is a classic symptom of yellow fever.

In fatal cases, the infection leads to kidney failure. The kidneys are responsible for maintaining the purity of body fluids and expelling wastes from the body. Death due to serious infection usually occurs within ten to fourteen days after the first symptoms appear.

2

THE HISTORY OF YELLOW FEVER

Written accounts of yellow fever date back nearly three and a half centuries. These writings provide us with some understanding of past outbreaks and epidemics. Over the past 350 years, yellow fever has been the cause of major epidemics throughout the world. Repeated epidemics have occurred in Africa and in South and Central America. The disease has also caused outbreaks in North America, the Caribbean islands, and parts of Europe.

It is estimated that during the late 1600s and the 1700s, seven out of every ten cases of yellow fever resulted in death. Pinpointing the actual number of people affected by yellow fever throughout history is incredibly difficult, however. This is because before the 1900s, people reacted to illness with fear and panic. Outbreaks of illnesses sent otherwise organized towns and cities into utter chaos. Many people who feared illness fled from areas of outbreak, leaving responsibilities, loved ones, and family members behind. Accurate death records were difficult to keep under such conditions.

Incubation and Immunity

Yellow fever is a dangerous and often deadly disease. There are conditions, however, that can and have limited the devastation brought about by yellow fever epidemics. Two major conditions are the incubation period of the virus and the ability of humans to become immune to the disease. Researchers believe that both of these conditions can also help us to understand where the yellow fever virus originally came from.

Incubation Period

An incubation period is the amount of time that it takes for a virus to develop within its host. During this time, no symptoms of illness occur. It is only after the incubation period that a host or vector becomes infectious. When a host becomes infectious, it means that the host now has the ability to pass the illness on to others.

The incubation period of yellow fever in mosquitoes is anywhere from nine to twenty-one days after they bite an infected host. It is only after this period of time that the mosquito becomes infectious. This means that if the mosquito bites another host before the incubation period is over, no virus will be transmitted.

The same is true for humans and primates. After being bitten by an infectious mosquito, the virus has an incubation period of three to six days in humans, and two to five days in primates. At the point that symptoms start to show, there is a time frame of three to four days during which the person or primate is infectious to mosquitoes. The mosquito must bite the human or primate during this time in order to become infected itself.

Researchers and historians believe that without the limitations of this infectious period, the virus could have been much more devastating. The disease could have been spread far more quickly. This would have increased the number of people infected.

Immunity

When a person is immune to something, it means that he or she will not be affected by it. When a person is immune to yellow fever, he or she will not be infected with or suffer the effects of the virus.

1668–1691

In North America, epidemics strike New York, Philadelphia, and Boston.

1730

In Europe, a two-month-long epidemic results in 22,000 deaths.

1751

In Africa, an epidemic decimates the populations of Guinea's coast, Senegal, and West Africa.

1699

First epidemic hits Mexico.

1734

Epidemics ravage Albany, Boston, New York, and Philadelphia.

1830–1840

Florida is ravaged. Yellow fever causes a delay in Florida being named a state.

Immunity to the disease occurs under certain circumstances including past infection and constant exposure to the virus.

When a person has been infected with yellow fever and recovers, he or she will now be immune and will not get the disease again. This is a lifelong immunity. Mothers can even pass along immunity to their newborns, which will protect infants for six months or longer.

There are also areas of the world where the virus occurs on a regular basis. People who live in these areas experience mild infection rather than serious infection. This is a mild immunity, or a resistance to

1878

An epidemic in the Mississippi region of North America is responsible for more than 20,000 deaths. Memphis, Tennessee, is nearly abandoned.

1900

In West Africa, the population of Dakar is almost entirely decimated.

1984–1993

In Africa, more than 20,000 cases in Nigeria result in over 4,000 deaths.

1960–1962

In Africa, Ethiopia experiences the largest outbreak ever recorded, resulting in 30,000 deaths.

1995

In Peru, South America, one-third of 440 cases result in death.

the disease. This natural resistance is brought about by regular exposure to the virus. It's one of the ways that yellow fever has been and is prevented from becoming a full-scale epidemic in certain areas of the world.

The Controversy over the Origin of Yellow Fever

Scientists and researchers believe that yellow fever originated either in South America or in Africa. Both the incubation period and immunity play a role in determining the real origin of the disease. Scientists and researchers use these two factors in their studies.

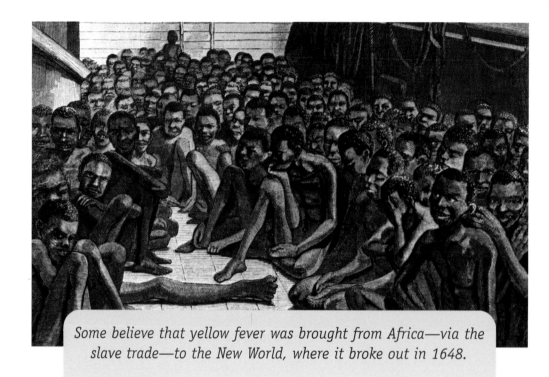

Some believe that yellow fever was brought from Africa—via the slave trade—to the New World, where it broke out in 1648.

According to the World Health Organization, the first account of yellow fever in South America occurred in 1648, and the first account of yellow fever in Africa occurred in 1768. Despite the fact that the first recorded illness occurred in South America, many researchers believe that the virus originally came from Africa.

Researchers base this belief on the fact that major epidemics occurred in South America in the years following 1648. This suggests that the people living in South America had no immunity to the disease at that time. This lack of immunity suggests that the virus was not present on the American continent until sometime around 1648.

Researchers believe that the disease was brought to the Americas by slave ships from Africa. Modern immunity patterns also show that humans and primates from Africa are more immune to yellow fever than are humans and primates from South and Central America. This suggests that the inhabitants of Africa have a longer history of exposure to yellow fever than do Americans.

Making the Leap

The slave trade from Africa to the Americas had been taking place for 100 years prior to 1648. Supporters of the African origin theory believe it may have taken this amount of time for the yellow fever virus to finally make its way across the Atlantic. In order for the virus to survive the voyage, certain conditions had to be just right. Decades would have passed before the right conditions took place at the same time.

Slave ships took an average of ten to twelve weeks to cross the Atlantic from Africa to the Americas. If the crew of the ship became infected prior to boarding, this voyage was long enough for victims to die or to survive and develop an immunity. In these circumstances, the virus would not have been able to survive the voyage. In order for the virus to survive on the ship for this amount of time, crew members would have needed to be infected at different points throughout the voyage. This means that vectors (mosquitoes) would have to have been present on the ship. If a crew member was infected by a mosquito bite just prior to arrival in the Americas, the disease could have been transmitted to the population.

The Stranger's Disease

Throughout the seventeenth and eighteenth centuries, Europeans who traveled to certain areas in Africa and the Americas were in great danger of catching the yellow fever virus. This is because they had no immunity to the disease. They had no immunity because they had never before been exposed to the virus. Because inhabitants of infected areas became relatively immune whereas newcomers fell victim to the virus almost immediately, yellow fever became known as the "stranger's disease."

Native inhabitants of the areas became wary of strangers because yellow fever activity increased upon their arrival. One such case occurred during the Irish immigration of the 1840s to New Orleans. In the 1850s, epidemics of yellow fever occurred throughout New Orleans and southern parts of the United States. The epidemics were blamed on the immigrants and their lack of immunity to the disease.

In 1655, France sent 1,500 soldiers to conquer the Caribbean islands. After exposure to and infection by the yellow fever virus at Saint Lucia, only eighty-nine of the soldiers survived. In 1741, Admiral Edward Vernon and 19,000 English soldiers were sent to Cartagena. Half of this force, around 9,500 soldiers, died after exposure to and infection by the virus. In 1802, France sent 25,000 soldiers to conquer Haiti. The troops became infected with yellow fever, and only 3,000 of the soldiers survived.

Massive death tolls like these earned certain areas of the world the nickname of "white man's grave." It was not until the early 1900s, when yellow fever vaccines were developed, that European travelers could safely travel to areas where yellow fever was present.

Efforts to Prevent Epidemics

Before 1900, the cause of yellow fever was not known. Some doctors believed that the disease came from the unsanitary and often filthy conditions in most cities and towns. Because there were no sewers, human and animal waste was not disposed of in a safe, clean way. Doctors believed that yellow fever came from the air that rose from dead animals and human and animal waste.

Doctors also thought that the disease was more likely to occur during hot weather. They believed that the hot weather heated the human waste and dead animals, which brought out the disease. Doctors ordered cleanups of dirty cities and towns in an effort to lower the risk of epidemics. The virus did occur more during the hot months of summer, but the increase in virus activity was not a result of heated waste. It was due to the fact that mosquitoes breed and are most active during the hot months of the year.

Doctors also relied on quarantines to keep yellow fever from spreading. A quarantine was a period of forty days and nights in which specific areas that contained infected persons were closed off. Ships were commonly subjected to quarantines. No one could enter or leave quarantined areas.

The quarantine was not a very successful practice for two reasons. Although the hosts could be held, the small, unsuspected mosquitoes, which were the real culprits behind the spread of the disease, could not be. Merchants were also frustrated with quarantines. Fruits, vegetables, and other foodstuffs often spoiled and rotted on quarantined ships. This left merchants without the goods that they desperately needed.

Making Progress in the Battle

In the second half of the 1800s, doctors and researchers began to suspect that there were possible causes of disease other than the traditionally accepted sources. The discovery of germs led doctors to take the focus off the world we see around us and place it on the world of the unseen. Researchers began looking for a germ that caused and spread yellow fever.

In a short time, several researchers were able to identify a yellow fever germ. It was soon discovered, however, that the germs themselves did not cause the spread of the disease. Something else was spreading yellow fever.

Doctor Walter Reed

In 1899, the United States surgeon general sent a team of researchers to Cuba to study yellow fever. Doctor Walter Reed was chosen to head the team. Reed decided to test a theory that the disease was not spread by a germ, but rather by mosquitoes.

Historians believe that Reed was set on his path to discovery by two different possible factors. One was the fact that research was being conducted on the cause of another disease called malaria. At the time that Dr. Reed was testing his theory, it had already been proposed in the medical community that malaria was spread by mosquitoes. In 1897, research about malaria and mosquitoes had been released by a British army doctor named Ronald Ross.

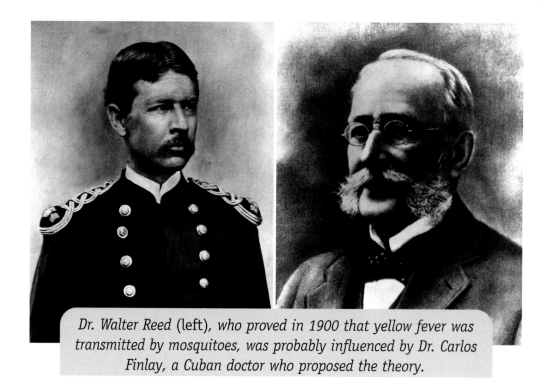

Dr. Walter Reed (left), who proved in 1900 that yellow fever was transmitted by mosquitoes, was probably influenced by Dr. Carlos Finlay, a Cuban doctor who proposed the theory.

The other possible factor that directed Dr. Reed's research was the writings of a Cuban doctor by the name of Carlos Finlay. In 1881, Finlay had published a paper in which he proposed that yellow fever was transmitted by mosquitoes. Many members of the community thought that his idea was the answer to what was spreading the disease.

In September 1900, Dr. Reed proved without doubt that yellow fever was transmitted by mosquitoes. To test his theory, Dr. Reed used two groups of volunteer soldiers who were quarantined under different circumstances. One group was placed in a house filled with patients infected by yellow fever—along with their

- Mosquitoes carry diseases such as yellow fever, encephalitis, heartworm, and malaria.
- There are over 3,000 different types, or species, of mosquitoes.
- Mosquitoes are cold-blooded.
- Only female mosquitoes bite humans in order to get protein, which is necessary for breeding and laying eggs.
- Mosquitoes do not bite in temperatures below 50 degrees.
- The life span of the average mosquito is two to three months.
- Mosquitoes that hibernate can live for as long as six to eight months.

filthy blankets and clothing, which were often covered with vomit and blood. The second group of volunteer soldiers was placed in a clean house where they were exposed to mosquitoes that had bitten yellow fever patients. Only the mosquito-bitten soldiers developed yellow fever.

3

YELLOW FEVER TODAY

Despite modern medical and preventative measures, yellow fever outbreaks and epidemics still occur today. The World Health Organization (WHO) estimates that the virus causes 30,000 deaths per year.

Today, yellow fever occurs mainly in Africa and Central and South America. In these areas, the virus usually causes mild infections within small populations. It is, however, capable of triggering outbreaks. Outbreaks in Africa can infect hundreds of thousands of people.

In addition to Africa and South and Central America, there are other areas of the world that are at risk for yellow fever. In fact, any area of the world where yellow fever has occurred in the past is still considered an area

- Baltimore—seven epidemics
- Boston—eight epidemics
- Philadelphia—twenty epidemics
- New York—fifteen epidemics
- New Orleans—more than twenty-three epidemics

of possible outbreak in the future. This includes many large cities in the United States, such as New Orleans and Memphis.

The Threat of Yellow Fever

According to WHO, the total number of yellow fever infections over the last twenty years has increased rather than decreased. There have also been a number of cases reported in countries where yellow fever does not usually occur. There are a few factors that may be playing a part in the growing number of yellow fever cases.

WHO estimates that mosquito populations and mosquito breeding grounds are increasing. An increase in the mosquito population can often lead to an increase in yellow fever activity. There are also large numbers of people throughout the world who are not yet immune to yellow fever. A lack of immunity is always a dangerous situation, as immunity is one of the main factors that will limit the threat of a disease. The increasing waves of deforestation (cutting down of forests) and urbanization (building cities in deforested areas) are also factors in increased yellow fever activity. Both these practices bring humans and infected mosquitoes into more frequent contact. Finally, the convenience and speed of world travel may make it easier for yellow fever to spread over vast distances.

Yellow Fever in South America—A Persistent Problem

Yellow fever infection in South America takes place in areas covered by tropical forests. Many of the infections take place among people who work in or near the forests. Forest workers and agricultural laborers working newly cleared land are at the greatest risk for exposure. According to WHO, about 80 percent of all yellow fever cases in South America take place among forest workers. These

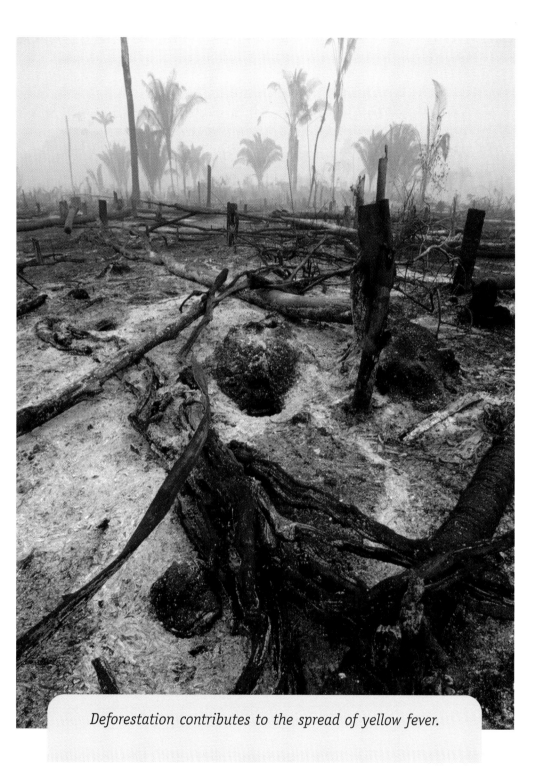

Deforestation contributes to the spread of yellow fever.

people are infected when they become a part of the natural cycle of jungle transmission in the wild.

In the past fifty years, many countries in South America have taken measures to eradicate the yellow fever virus. In 1949, a group of ten South and Central American countries mounted a massive campaign to wipe out the *Aedes aegypti* mosquito. Efforts were focused on destroying mosquito breeding grounds.

By 1954, Brazil had wiped out its entire population of *Aedes aegypti* mosquitoes. By 1965, a large portion of the mosquito population had been removed from most of the urban areas of South and Central America. As a result of the mosquito removal, yellow fever activity declined, and the efforts seemed to be paying off. In the years following the massive campaign, however, the mosquitoes returned to their old breeding grounds.

WHO estimates that over 100 cases of yellow fever still occur yearly in Brazil, Colombia, Ecuador, and Peru. These countries are still at risk for potential outbreaks as well. In 1995, Peru experienced a jungle transmission outbreak in which more than one-third of 440 reported cases resulted in death.

Africa, Then and Now

Between 1927 and 1931, the number of yellow fever cases in Africa was on the decline. The virus seemed

Just prior to 1990, a new mosquito vector was discovered in South America. The *Aedes albopictus*, which came to the Americas from Asia, was found to be a strong vector of the yellow fever virus. The *Aedes albopictus* now inhabits a zone between urban and forest areas. The mosquito is poised to cause more outbreaks in human and primate populations.

to be disappearing from one area after another. It seemed as if Africa was well on its way to freeing itself from the dreaded disease. Then, suddenly, in 1931, multiple outbreaks exploded across many different areas of the continent.

Researchers explain the sudden increase in virus activity as a result of the fact that the virus had been laying dormant, or inactive, for a few years prior to 1931. When the virus became active again, the results were devastating. A large number of the victims were Europeans who had recently settled in Africa. The Europeans did not have prior exposure to the virus and had no immunity.

Efforts were made to discover which factors had brought about additional epidemics in Africa. It was discovered that forestry practices had played a large part in spreading the disease. As trees were cut down, mosquitoes that had been dwelling in the treetops were brought down to the ground. This brought humans and mosquitoes closer together. In addition to the effects of deforestation, studies that took place in Nigeria during the 1970s proved that in addition to *Aedes aegypti*, the common *Aedes africanus* mosquito was also acting as a vector in urban transmission.

Waging War Against the Fever

Efforts have been made to control epidemics in Africa. Monkeys have been hunted, which has decreased the number of jungle hosts, and mosquito breeding grounds have been destroyed. Even with these efforts, conditions still exist that are favorable for the spread of the disease. Overpopulation in some areas contributes to a large supply of hosts for the disease. Water sources created in areas populated by humans also provide prime breeding grounds for mosquitoes.

Main Areas of Yellow Fever Activity

Outbreaks of yellow fever in Africa occur in three main areas: the humid savannah, the dry savannah, and the rain forests near the equator. Virus activity is greatest in the humid savannah.

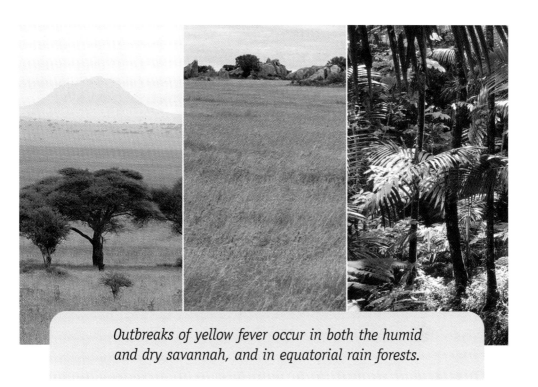

Outbreaks of yellow fever occur in both the humid and dry savannah, and in equatorial rain forests.

The humid savannah area makes up parts of West and Central Africa. During the rainy seasons, this area experiences increased yellow fever activity. This is an area with high numbers of both hosts and vectors.

The dry savannah makes up part of Central and North Africa and includes countries such as Senegal. Explosive outbreaks can occur if the virus is introduced to urban areas of the dry savannah. In these areas, the human populations store water, which is then used as breeding grounds for the *Aedes aegypti* mosquitoes. Explosive yellow fever outbreaks can spread from village to village through the travel of hosts or vectors.

The equatorial rain forest area includes the countries of Guinea, Uganda, Equatorial Guinea, and Angola. Angola experiences year-round yellow fever activity. Yellow fever occurs periodically in the other areas of the equatorial rain forest.

Big Risk in Africa

To this day, Africa is at great risk for major yellow fever epidemics. There is a population of 468 million people in Africa who live in areas of yellow fever activity. In addition, many of these people live in countries that have very few medical professionals and little medical equipment. This further increases the risk of epidemics.

4

DIAGNOSIS AND TREATMENT

A diagnosis is the determination of an illness in a patient. A doctor must follow a number of procedures to diagnose an illness correctly. The very first step in diagnosing an illness is to examine the symptoms. Symptoms are signs of disease or illness. Some symptoms are shared by different illnesses. Since yellow fever shares symptoms with other diseases, diagnosing yellow fever can be difficult.

Illnesses such as dengue fever, ebola fever, hepatitis, influenza, malaria, mononucleosis, rickets, and typhoid have symptoms similar to yellow fever. Some symptoms of yellow fever also resemble common symptoms of poisoning. Shared symptoms include a sudden onset of sickness, general aches, and vomiting. Because yellow fever has so many shared symptoms, doctors rely on further medical procedures to rule out other illnesses. The most useful procedure in confirming yellow fever infection is the blood test.

Testing for Yellow Fever

A blood test will detect whether a host's body is producing antibodies. Antibodies are produced within the body in order to attack foreign substances such as viruses and bacteria. During yellow fever infection, the body of the host will produce antibodies that are specially designed to attack only yellow fever virions. These antibodies usually appear by the third or fourth day of infection.

Other blood tests can locate yellow fever virus particles in the blood. The virus particles can be found in the blood during the first three to four days of infection. After this time, the viruses are more difficult to locate.

Tests can also be performed on patients who died with yellow fever–like symptoms but who were never formally diagnosed. A common test of this type is the liver biopsy. A tissue specimen is taken from the liver and analyzed. The tissue sample can reveal if the patient died of yellow fever.

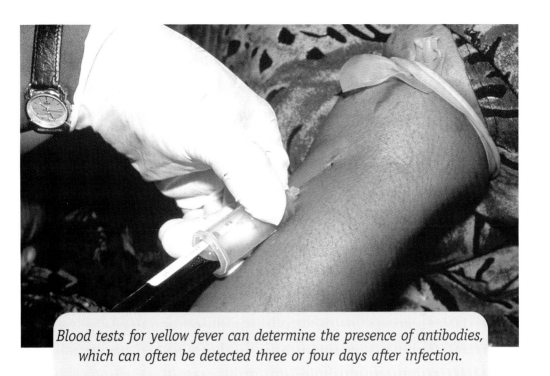

Blood tests for yellow fever can determine the presence of antibodies, which can often be detected three or four days after infection.

Highly trained laboratory staff and specialized equipment are required for blood and tissue testing. Strict procedures must be followed in obtaining blood and tissue samples, or the results may be inaccurate. Samples must also be labeled, packed, and transported correctly.

Symptoms of Yellow Fever

According to the Centers for Disease Control and Prevention (CDC), there are two stages of yellow fever infection during which common symptoms occur.

These stages are mild infection and classic yellow fever (severe infection). In both stages, the virus causes no symptoms during the first three to six days. During this time, the virus is incubating, or developing inside of the human host. After the incubation period is over, symptoms start to appear.

Mild Infection

A mild infection of yellow fever is less dangerous than classic, or severe, yellow fever. After symptoms first appear, mild infections usually run their course in three to four days. At this point, most patients improve and the symptoms disappear.

Common symptoms of mild yellow fever infection include back and muscle pains, bradycardia (an abnormally slow heart rate that can cause dizziness, fainting, fatigue, and shortness of breath), chills, congestion, skin flushing (reddening of skin on the face and neck), headache, fever (100 degrees or higher), nausea, vomiting, loss of appetite, possible bleeding from the mouth, and reddening of the tongue.

Severe Infection—Classic Yellow Fever

According to the CDC, about 20 to 50 percent of all severe yellow fever infections are fatal. The surviving patients will eventually return to normal and will

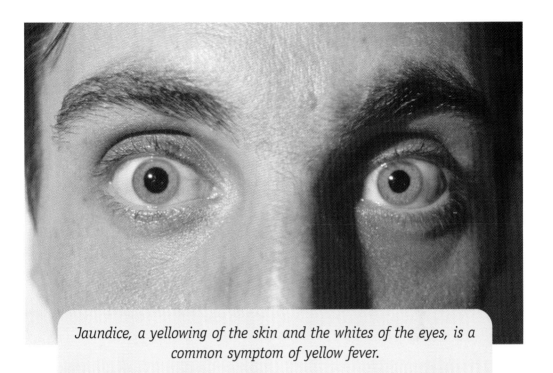

Jaundice, a yellowing of the skin and the whites of the eyes, is a common symptom of yellow fever.

have sustained little or no damage to their organs as a result of the infection.

Patients who develop severe infections will experience a short period of time where the infection subsides. During this time—one to three days—the patient is relieved from the effects of the symptoms. After this period, the infection symptoms return and can progress to a deadly outcome.

Common symptoms of classic yellow fever including abdominal pain, fever, jaundice (yellowing of the skin and the whites of the eyes), vomiting of blood, dehydration (lack of fluids in the body), abnormal liver function, abnormal kidney function, and absolute exhaustion.

In addition to these symptoms, there are further symptoms that increase the possibility of death within ten to fourteen days of infection. These symptoms include brain disease (encephalopathy—causing disorientation and confusion), deepened jaundice, hemorrhaging (bleeding from the eyes, mouth, nose, rectum, or stomach), liver failure, kidney failure, and shock.

Treatment of Yellow Fever

Some illnesses caused by germs can be cured with medicine. Most viruses, however, cannot be cured by the use of medicine. While ill with yellow fever, patients may experience other infections that are caused by bacteria. These infections can be treated with medicine, but the drugs have no effect on the yellow fever virus itself.

Doctors may also prescribe drugs that help to relieve some of the symptoms that are caused by yellow fever infection. Symptoms such as fever and dehydration are treated with drugs such as paracetamol and rehydration salts. In areas where it is available, patients with severe infection and symptoms are given intensive care.

For treatment of all yellow fever infection, doctors order infected patients to drink plenty of liquids and to rest. Patients are also placed in locations where they will not be bitten by mosquitoes. After a long period of rest and care, some patients may completely recover.

Because there are no cures for the actual yellow fever infection, doctors and researchers place a great deal of emphasis on disease prevention and control. Through the prevention and control of yellow fever, fewer people are infected. This means that there are fewer people in need of a medicine that doesn't exist.

5

PREVENTION AND CONTROL

In 1901, shortly after Dr. Walter Reed proved that mosquitoes were responsible for spreading yellow fever, Dr. William Crawford Gorgas set out to control the mosquito populations in certain yellow fever–bearing areas. He focused his efforts first in Havana, Cuba, and later in the area that had been set aside for the construction of the Panama Canal.

Gorgas lowered the amount of adult mosquitoes in these areas by draining pools of standing water and by using insecticides. Having less water around cut down on the breeding grounds for mosquitoes. The insecticides killed mosquitoes outright.

Gorgas was successful in practically eliminating yellow fever by controlling the mosquito populations. His work proved that by controlling mosquito populations, yellow fever epidemics could be avoided.

Mosquito Control

Today, measures are taken to control the mosquito population in areas where the virus exists or could occur. The main mode of control is eliminating mosquito breeding sites in and near urban centers. By eliminating extra or unused water sources, the mosquito population is effectively lowered. In addition, insecticides are used to kill mosquitoes during outbreaks and epidemics.

To control jungle mosquitoes, aerial spraying is necessary. Aerial spraying is done by planes that drop, or dust, large amounts of poisons over an area. Spraying for jungle mosquitoes is very impractical because the areas to be covered are vast and the cost of aerial spraying is very high. In addition, most insecticides used in aerial spraying are also harmful to humans, animals, and the environment. In the case of jungle mosquitoes, we must attempt to limit our exposure to them or to increase our immunity to the disease.

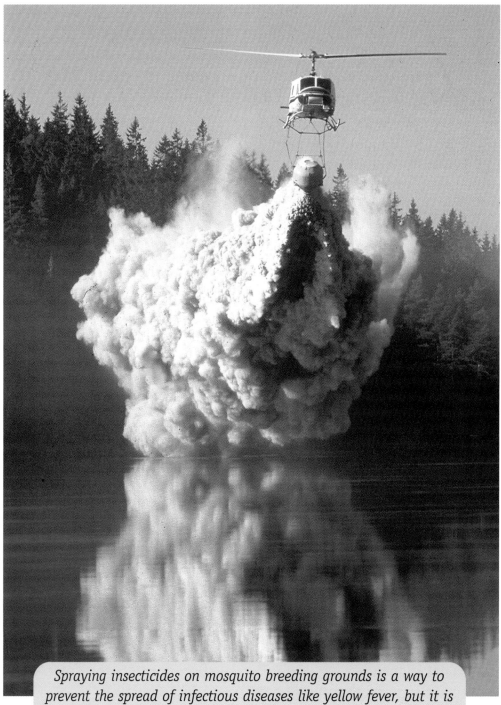

Spraying insecticides on mosquito breeding grounds is a way to prevent the spread of infectious diseases like yellow fever, but it is usually impractical.

Who's at Risk?

According to the CDC, anyone is at risk of contracting yellow fever who travels to areas where yellow fever has infected humans, primates, or vector mosquitoes. There have been reports of travelers and tourists who died because of yellow fever infection. An area is considered to be at risk if the area:

- Has a history of yellow fever outbreaks and epidemics
- Has inhabitants who are exposed to forests or jungles where yellow fever exists
- Has the types of mosquitoes that can spread the virus
- Has a long rainy season
- Is often traveled by inhabitants from yellow fever areas
- Is near forested or jungle areas with large primate populations

Vaccines—the Best Prevention

The discovery of viruses in the early 1900s prompted research into creating medicines that would treat or

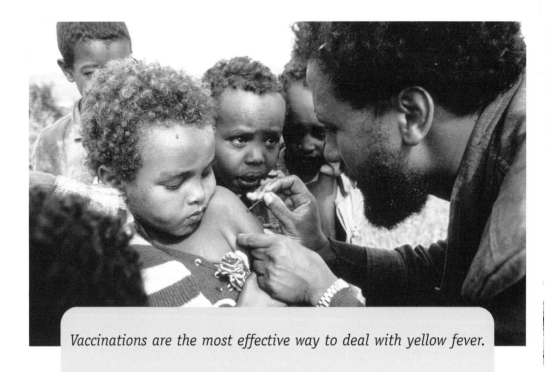

Vaccinations are the most effective way to deal with yellow fever.

prevent illnesses. This research led to the creation of vaccines. A vaccine is a medicine that, when administered, or given, provides immunity to a particular disease. When a person is given a vaccine, it is called a vaccination.

The use of a yellow fever vaccine can render a person immune. This means that after receiving a vaccine for yellow fever, a person will be immune to the disease. He or she will not become infected with the disease, even after being exposed to the virus. Yellow fever vaccines have been used for more than sixty years. Most vaccines are administered in liquid form through a syringe, or needle.

The yellow fever vaccine is given to anyone who is considered to be at risk for becoming infected. Vaccinations are given to anyone that will have contact with infected areas or infected people. Travelers going to infected areas receive vaccinations before traveling to those areas. Many countries with a history of yellow fever epidemics will not allow entry unless travelers show proof that they have received the vaccination. People who live in areas where the virus maintains a natural cycle are also given vaccinations.

Yellow Fever Immunization

There are a few different types of vaccines for yellow fever. The most used vaccine is called 17-D. It also happens to be the least expensive, which is a very important factor in many countries of Africa and South America where there are economic and financial troubles.

The 17-D vaccination, which was developed in the 1930s, is very effective and safe to use. A single dose of 17-D will protect an adult for life. Children under four years old who are vaccinated are protected for at least ten years from the day of vaccination. The vaccination can be given to children as young as nine months old. It takes about seven days after the vaccination for immunity to develop.

According to WHO, over three hundred million vaccinations have been given. Routine vaccinations are done on a regular basis regardless of epidemic threat. This ensures that if the virus infects some members of the population, almost everyone else will already be immune. People who receive these vaccinations experience few side effects or reactions to the medication.

In the case of large epidemics, massive emergency immunization campaigns are used. Emergency vaccinations are less effective than routine vaccinations. This is due to the fact that, under emergency conditions, recently immunized members could still be infected while waiting for the vaccination to work (seven days after getting the vaccination). People who received a routine immunization are already immune in the event of an epidemic.

Surveillance

According to the CDC, yellow fever is a preventable disease. The most important steps to prevent the transmission of the disease to humans are mosquito control and immunization. Another important step, surveillance, can keep yellow fever infections from turning into epidemics. Surveillance is carefully watching, or watching for, someone or something.

Most large epidemics of yellow fever are already under way by the time that the virus is recognized as the cause. The CDC states that many deaths and cases of yellow fever infection can be prevented by close surveillance in areas with a history of epidemics or virus and vector activity.

Surveillance isolates the virus before it can reach and infect more people. According to the CDC, the best way to prevent epidemics is to recognize mild infections as early as possible. Any suspected infections are to be reported to state health departments, the CDC, or WHO.

Organizations such as the World Health Organization and the Centers for Disease Control and Prevention are researching ways of getting aid to areas of need in Africa and South America. Organizations such as these are also monitoring the possible vector mosquito populations in areas where the disease has struck before, such as America.

An Ever-Present Danger

Although the tropics are the areas most at risk for yellow fever infection, conditions exist in the United States that could lead to outbreaks. The *Aedes aegypti* mosquito can survive the winters of the United States as far north as Memphis,

Tennessee. In the face of this continuing danger, health organizations continue to be vigilant in their surveillance of the disease.

GLOSSARY

antibodies Substances made by the body to attack foreign substances.

carcass The body of a dead animal.

deforestation The cutting down of forests.

epidemic An outbreak of disease in a human population.

germ A microorganism; a very tiny, living thing.

hemorrhaging The discharging of blood in large amounts.

immunization The practice of vaccination.

incubation A period of development or growth under favorable conditions.

infected Having a disease.

microorganism A tiny organism.

microscope A device with a curved piece of glass, called a lens, that makes small things look larger.

organism Any living thing.

surveillance Carefully watching something or watching for something.

transmission Spread of disease from one source to another.

urbanization The building of cities in deforested or wild and rural areas.

vaccination The administering of a vaccine.

vaccine A medicine that provides immunity to a disease.

vector An insect or organism that carries and transmits disease.

virion An individual virus particle.

virus A germ that causes disease.

FOR MORE INFORMATION

In the United States

Centers for Disease Control and Prevention (CDC)
National Center for Infectious Diseases
1600 Clifton Road
Atlanta, GA 30333
(800) 311-3435
Web site: http://www.cdc.gov

The World Health Organization (WHO)
    Regional Office for the Americas/Pan American
Health Organization (AMRO/PAHO)
525 23rd Street NW
Washington, DC 20037
(202) 974-3000
e-mail: postmaster@paho.org
Web site: http://www.paho.org

In Canada

Health Canada—General Inquiries
A.L. 0904A
Ottawa, ON K1A 0K9
(613) 957-2991

Health Canada—Quebec
Room 218, Complexe Guy-Favreau, East Tower
200 René Lévesque Boulevard, West
Montreal, QC H2Z 1X4
(514) 283-2306

Health Canada—Toronto
25 Saint Clair Avenue East, 4th Floor
Toronto, ON M4T 1M2
(416) 973-4389

FOR FURTHER READING

Anderson, Laurie Halse. *Fever 1793*. New York: Simon
& Schuster, 2000.

Berger, Melvin, and Marylin Hafner. *Germs Make Me
Sick!* (Lets-Read-And-Find-Out Science). New
York: Harper Trophy, 1995.

Facklam, Howard, and Margery Facklam. *Viruses*
(Invaders). Breckenridge, CO: Twenty-First
Century Books, 1995.

Holley, Dennis. *Viruses and Bacteria: Hands-On
Minds-On Activities for Middle School and High
School*. Pacific Grove, CA: Critical Thinking Books
and Software, 1999.

Marsh, Carole. *Hot Zones: Diseases, Epidemics,
Viruses and Bacteria*. Peachtree City, GA:
Gallopade Publishing Group, 1998.

Nourse, Alan. *The Virus Invaders*. Danbury, CT:
Franklin Watts, 1992.

INDEX

CREDITS

About the Author

Holly Cefrey is a writer and researcher in New York. She has authored a number of books about diseases, including the plague, cancer, and AIDS.

Photo Credits

Series Design

Evelyn Horovicz

Layout

Thomas Forget